I0841631

Understanding and Overcoming Metabolic Syndrome: A Comprehensive Guide to Health

By

Badmus Owolabi

Table of Contents

Copyright © Bailey Holt 2023. All rights reserved

Before this document is duplicated or reproduced in any manner, the publisher's consent must be gained.

Therefore, the contents within can neither be stored electronically, transferred, nor kept in a database. Neither in part nor in full can the document be copied, scanned, faxed, or retained without approval from the publisher or creator.

Introduction

The danger metabolic syndrome (MetS) carries for heart disease, type 2 diabetes, and other dangerous illnesses such as nonalcoholic fatty liver disease makes it very important. This book reviews the scientific literature to provide advice for managing and preventing MetS, including lifestyle modifications and their components. MetS can be prevented and treated partly by losing weight through an energy-restricted diet and increasing energy expenditure through physical activity.

An efficient part of treatment is a Mediterranean-style diet, with or without energy restriction. The foundation of this dietary pattern should be an increase in unsaturated fat, mostly from olive oil. It should also place a strong emphasis on the consumption of low-fat dairy products, legumes, cereals, fruits, vegetables, nuts, fish, and cereals, as well as modest amounts of alcohol. There have also been suggestions for other dietary regimens (Dietary Approaches to Stop Hypertension, new Nordic diets, and vegetarian diets) as alternatives for preventing MetS. It is essential to give up smoking and cut back on meat and meat products, as well as sugar-sweetened beverages.

There are also misunderstandings and lapses in the data; therefore, more findings are required to determine the best treatments for MetS. A healthy maintenance lifestyle is important to preventing or stopping the onset of MetS in those who are in it, as well as preventing type 2 diabetes and cardiovascular disease in those who already have MetS. This book's recommendations should aid in the understanding and application of the best lifestyle modification strategies for improving cardiometabolic health and preventing MetS by patients and doctors. If lifestyle modifications are insufficient to manage the diseases associated with metabolic syndrome, your healthcare provider may recommend medication to decrease blood pressure, cholesterol, and other symptoms. Adhering to the instructions provided by your healthcare team can aid in averting numerous chronic consequences of metabolic syndrome. Your health will improve as a result of your diligence and focus in these areas.

I present this to you as the source of inspiration for the work included inside these pages, which comprises guided prescriptions and practices to help you navigate through your deepest state of health. Get into a permanent state of health; every action matters.

Chapter 1: What is Metabolic Syndrome?

The main cause of metabolic syndrome, a complicated condition with several risk factors, is insulin resistance along with abnormal adipose deposition and function. It consists of a mix of risk factors for diabetes, fatty liver, several malignancies, and coronary heart disease. These conditions include hypertension, hyperglycemia, adiposity around the waist, and hypercholesterolemia or hypertriglyceridemia.

Another way to categorize metabolic syndrome is as one of five conditions that have the potential to cause heart disease, diabetes, stroke, and other health issues. When three or more of these risk factors are present, metabolic syndrome is diagnosed. Even if just one of them raises the risk of cardiovascular disease, the likelihood of having a major cardiovascular condition increases if a person has three or more of these risk factors and is diagnosed with metabolic syndrome. For instance, abdominal obesity (having a big waistline) and high fasting blood sugar levels increase the risk of cardiovascular disease. High blood pressure is a significant risk factor for cardiovascular disease; physical inactivity, overweight and obesity, insulin resistance, hereditary factors, and aging are among the causes of metabolic syndrome.

A heart-healthy diet rich in whole grains, fruits, vegetables, and fish can lower your risk of developing metabolic syndrome, a serious condition for which there is no known cure. Work with your healthcare team to monitor and manage your blood pressure, blood glucose, and blood cholesterol. The disorders that make up metabolic syndrome raise your risk of stroke, type 2 diabetes, and cardiovascular disease. It can also result in illnesses including organ damage and atherosclerosis, which are disorders linked to plaque accumulation in arterial walls. Insulin resistance syndrome, syndrome X, and dysmetabolic syndrome are among the other names for metabolic syndrome.

Chapter 2: *Signs and Symptoms of Metabolic Syndrome*

The majority of metabolic syndrome-related illnesses lack overt symptoms or indicators. A noticeable indicator is a big waist circumference. Additionally, if your blood sugar level is high, you may have fatigue, impaired vision, increased thirst and urination, and other symptoms of diabetes. Individuals with metabolic syndrome usually have larger waists and a lot of weight around their abdomens, giving them an apple-shaped body type. It is believed that having a pear-shaped body—that is, putting more weight on your hips and having a smaller waist—does not put you at higher risk of developing diabetes, heart disease, or other metabolic syndrome-related problems.

You do not automatically have metabolic syndrome if you only have one of these disorders. However, it does increase your chance of developing a serious illness. Additionally, your risk of complications like type 2 diabetes and heart disease increases even further if you have more of these disorders. The prevalence of metabolic syndrome is rising, with up to one-third of adult Americans suffering from it. Aggressive lifestyle modifications can postpone or even stop the onset of major health issues if you have metabolic syndrome or any of its components.

Heart disease, stroke, and type 2 diabetes are all made more likely by the group of disorders known as metabolic syndrome. These disorders include hypertension, hyperglycemia, adiposity around the waist, and elevated triglyceride or cholesterol levels.

Apple and pear body shapes

An individual with metabolic syndrome usually has larger waists and a lot of weight around their abdomens, giving them an apple-shaped body type. It is believed that having a pear-shaped body—that is, putting more weight on your hips and having a smaller waist—does not put you at higher risk of developing diabetes, heart disease, or other metabolic syndrome-related problems.

Chapter 3: Causes of Metabolic Syndrome

Being overweight, obese, and inactive are strongly associated with metabolic syndrome; it's connected to a disorder known as insulin resistance. Normally, the food you consume is broken down into sugar by your digestive system. Your pancreas secretes the hormone insulin, which facilitates the entry of sugar into your cells for use as fuel. Insulin resistance impairs a person's ability to allow glucose to enter cells and causes abnormal cell responses to insulin.

Consequently, even though your body is producing more and more insulin in an attempt to lower your blood sugar, your blood sugar levels continue to climb. The development of metabolic syndrome is caused by a complicated network of interrelated elements. However, scientists believe that the primary cause of the condition is insulin resistance. A complicated network of interrelated elements can lead to

diabetes. Hyperinsulinemia and insulin resistance can also be linked to:

- Obesity.
- Fatty liver disease.
- Polycystic ovary syndrome (PCOS).

The following can all contribute to insulin resistance:

- Obesity, or excess weight around the abdomen:

According to studies, having too much body fat, especially around the abdomen, raises your chance of developing insulin resistance. More visceral fat, or fat around your organs, than subcutaneous fat, or fat under your skin, contributes to insulin resistance. However, they are both involved in the metabolic syndrome.

- Absence of exercise: In order to operate, your muscles need a lot of glucose and glycogen, which is stored glucose. Engaging in physical activity increases insulin sensitivity and develops muscle that has a higher blood glucose absorption capacity. Conversely, inactivity can lead to insulin resistance and other negative consequences.

- Certain drugs: A number of drugs, including corticosteroids, blood pressure pills, several HIV medicines, and some psychiatric drugs, can result in insulin resistance.
- Genetics: The genes you inherited from your

biological parents can make you resistant to insulin. Additionally, they may be a factor in excessive blood pressure, high cholesterol, and obesity.

Chapter 4: Risk factors of Metabolic Syndrome

Knowing your risk factors for any disease can help guide you in taking the appropriate actions. This includes changing behaviors and being monitored by your healthcare provider for the disease. Certain factors—like your lifestyle choices and age or family history—affect your risk of metabolic syndrome, while other factors are beyond your control.

Risk variables are under your control.

The lifestyle choices listed below may increase your risk of developing metabolic syndrome.

1. Consuming large amounts of food and a poor diet.
2. Not receiving enough restorative sleep, which is important for regulating how well your body absorbs nutrients from meals.

3. Smoking and heavy alcohol consumption.

4. Occupation: Due to their frequently misaligned circadian clocks with their surroundings, shift workers are more susceptible to metabolic syndrome. This may result in issues with the body's ability to absorb nutrients from a diet.

Risky variables that you might not be able to manage

1. Age: As you age, you have a higher chance of developing metabolic syndrome.

2. Environment: Living in poverty can result in bad eating habits, a sedentary lifestyle, and inadequate sleep (sleep deprivation).

3. Genetics and family history: Your weight and the way your body reacts to insulin might be influenced by your genes. If any member of your family has ever had diabetes, metabolic syndrome, or any of its risk factors, you are more likely to get the condition yourself.

4. Nationality. Metabolic syndrome is more common in

Mexican Americans and African Americans. The illness affects African-American women almost 60% more frequently than African-American men.

5. BMI (body mass index) of more than 25. Body fat is measured using the BMI in relation to height and weight.

6. Diabetes in one's family or on oneself? Individuals who have a family member with type 2 diabetes or women who have experienced gestational diabetes during pregnancy are more

susceptible to metabolic syndrome.

7. Consuming tobacco
8. A past of binge drinking
9. Tensile
10. Passed the menopause
11. Fat-filled diet
12. Sedentary kind of life

Additional Medical Issues

The primary risk factors for metabolic syndrome are being overweight or obese, as these conditions can drop good high-density lipoprotein cholesterol and increase blood triglycerides, blood pressure, and bad low-density lipoprotein cholesterol. The risk of metabolic syndrome in your unborn child increases if you are overweight or obese during pregnancy.

Low birth weight and fast weight growth after delivery can increase an infant's chance of developing metabolic syndrome in later life. Having a wide waistline, high blood sugar, high triglyceride levels, and low levels of good cholesterol (high density lipoprotein), PCOS is caused by hormonal abnormalities in the body. Immune system issues can increase your risk of developing certain skin conditions, like psoriasis. You run a higher risk if you receive some cancer treatments that compromise your immune system.

Sleep issues, such as insufficient sleep, can increase your risk.

Certain medications used to treat schizophrenia, bipolar illness, depression, allergies, and HIV can increase your risk.

Sex: Women are more likely than men to develop metabolic syndrome as they age. This is due to the fact that hormonal changes that occur following menopause may increase the risk of excessive blood sugar, a large waist circumference, and low levels of healthy HDL cholesterol.

Chapter 5: Lifestyle recommendations for the prevention and management of metabolic syndrome

The circumstances that lead to metabolic syndrome may be avoided with a lifetime dedication to a healthy lifestyle. In order to treat metabolic syndrome, multiple problems must be addressed. This is what you can do as of right now:

- Eat more healthfully: Make whole grains,

fruits, vegetables, fish, nuts, skinless chicken, low-fat or fat-free dairy products, lean meats, and veggie protein a major part of your diet.

- Reduce your intake of processed foods, red meat, trans and saturated fats, sodium, and added sweets.

- Take action: Aim for 150 minutes or more per week of moderate-intense exercise. The simplest way to start is with walking, but you might also want to look for another activity you enjoy that raises your heart rate. To attain your goal, divide your exercise into multiple short periods spread throughout the day, if necessary.

- Get lighter.: You can lower your risk of heart disease by making weight-loss and maintenance changes. Find out how many calories you should be eating, how many calories you are burning off while you exercise at different levels, and your suggested calorie consumption. To achieve your objectives, strike a balance between a healthy diet and moderate activity.

- Giving up smoking: No smoking lowers the chance that the negative health impacts of metabolic syndrome will get worse.

Chapter 6: How is metabolic syndrome treated?

The optimal course of action for you will be determined by your healthcare professional, depending on:

- What is your age?
- How ill are you?
- How well you are able to manage particular medications, treatments, and procedures.
- How long is anticipated for the condition to persist.

Receiving therapy is crucial for metabolic syndrome since it raises the chance of acquiring more severe long-term (chronic) diseases. Type 2 diabetes and cardiovascular disease could develop if you don't get therapy. The following other ailments could arise PCOS, or polycystic ovarian syndrome.

- Gallstones, cholesterol, and fatty liver
- Airways
- Issues with sleep
- Certain types of cancer

The following are several kinds of treatments for metabolic

syndrome that may be suggested:

Lifestyle   ***Management***

Usually, treatment entails a change in lifestyle. This entails increasing your exercise, changing your diet under the guidance of a dietitian, and decreasing weight. Losing weight causes triglycerides and LDL ("bad") cholesterol to decrease and HDL ("good") cholesterol to rise. Additionally, reducing body weight can lower the incidence of type 2 diabetes. Even a small weight loss can reduce blood pressure and improve insulin sensitivity. Additionally, it might lessen the quantity of fat in your middle. Exercise, behavioral therapy, and diet reduce risk factors more than diet alone. Reducing your alcohol intake and giving up smoking are two more lifestyle adjustments.

Diet

Dietary modifications are crucial for the treatment of metabolic syndrome. Generally speaking, increasing physical activity and decreasing weight are the best ways to manage insulin resistance. To achieve this, take the following actions: Eat a wide range of foods in your diet. Employ good fats, Fats that are mono- and polyunsaturated may support heart health. Nuts, seeds, and some oils like canola, safflower, and olive include these good fats. Instead of white rice and white bread, choose whole grains like brown rice and whole-wheat bread. When it comes to nutrition, whole-grain foods are superior than highly processed ones. Because whole grains include more fiber, the body absorbs them more gradually. They don't result in an abrupt increase in insulin, which can lead to cravings and hunger. According to the USDA's 2015–2020 Dietary Guidelines, you should consume at least half of your grains as whole grains. When dining out, bring some of your food from the restaurant home. Ask for a take-home box when ordering takeout or dining out, and steer clear of super-size options. Think about splitting an entrée, as many restaurant portions are too big for one person. Alternatively, choose an appetizer from the entrée menu in place of a main course. Carefully read food labels. Take special note of the serving size and quantity of the product. If you consume the entire container of food, even if there are three servings per container and the label states that a serving is 150 calories, you will have consumed 450 calories. Select meals that don't have much-added sugar.

Exercise

Overweight and obese individuals benefit from exercise because it helps them maintain and gain lean body mass, or muscle tissue, while shedding fat. Because muscle tissue burns calories more quickly than non-muscular tissue, it also aids in weight loss more quickly than a good diet alone. Almost anybody can benefit greatly from walking as exercise. Begin gradually by going for a

30-minute walk several days a week. Increase the time gradually until you are walking for greater stretches of time most days of the week. Exercise can help prevent type 2 diabetes and reduce blood pressure. Along with these emotional benefits, exercise also lowers LDL cholesterol, decreases appetite, enhances flexibility, and improves sleep quality. Consult your physician before beginning any fitness regimen.

Medicine

Individuals with metabolic syndrome or those who are at risk for it may require medication as a form of treatment. This is particularly true if you have not seen any improvement from diet and other lifestyle modifications. Medication to assist lower blood pressure, enhance insulin metabolism, boost HDL cholesterol and decrease LDL cholesterol, promote weight loss, or any combination of these may be prescribed by your doctor.

Weight-loss surgery

If diet, exercise, or medication have not been successful in helping a patient lose weight, bariatric surgery, often known as weight-loss surgery, is an effective treatment for morbid obesity. It might also benefit those who are less fat but nonetheless experience serious health issues as a result of their obesity. Research indicates that a year following the procedure, blood pressure, cholesterol, and body weight were all reduced following gastric bypass surgery. Although there are various approaches to weight loss surgery, they are all malabsorptive, restrictive, or a mix of the two. The digestive system is altered by malabsorptive processes.

Procedures that significantly reduce stomach size are known as restrictive procedures. After then, the stomach may accommodate less food while still performing its digestive tasks.

Chapter 7: Conclusion

The first line of treatment and prevention for MetS is lifestyle modification. For those who are susceptible, maintaining a healthy lifestyle is essential to delaying or preventing the start of MetS. The suggestions made here ought to assist physicians and patients in comprehending and putting into practice the best lifestyle modification strategies in order to avoid MetS and enhance cardio-metabolic health.

The dietary pattern method, which more accurately captures the complexity of the interplay between several nutrients' effects on health, has replaced the single food approach in nutritional epidemiology research throughout the past ten years with regard to the dietary approach to prevention and treatment. This dietary pattern should be based on consuming more unsaturated fat, mainly from olive oil, and place emphasis on eating a range of foods, including cereals, legumes, fruits, vegetables, fish, nuts, and dairy products. It should also include moderate amounts of alcohol, such as red wine and/or beer.

In nutritional epidemiology research, the single food approach has been replaced over the past ten years with the dietary pattern method, which more accurately captures the complexity of the interplay between several nutrients' effects on health with regard to dietary prevention and treatment. This dietary pattern should emphasise eating a variety of foods, such as cereals, legumes, fruits, vegetables, seafood, nuts, and dairy products, and should be centred around ingesting more unsaturated fat, primarily from olive oil. Moderate amounts of alcohol, like red wine or beer, should also be included. The contradictions and gaps in the data presented here imply that more investigation is required to determine the best treatments for MetS.

www.ingramcontent.com/pod-product-compliance
Lightning Source LLC
Chambersburg PA
CBHW071003260726
48661CB00007B/2766